The Easy Way to Keeping Fit

Jane Bernard

AuthorHouse™ UK
1663 Liberty Drive
Bloomington, IN 47403 USA
www.authorhouse.co.uk
Phone: 0800.197.4150

Published by AuthorHouse 11/23/2016

ISBN: 978-1-5246-3541-1 (sc)
ISBN: 978-1-5246-3543-5 (e)

Print information available on the last page.

Any people depicted in stock imagery provided by Thinkstock are models,
and such images are being used for illustrative purposes only.
Certain stock imagery © Thinkstock.

This book is printed on acid-free paper.

Contents

DEDICATION

This work is dedicated to everyone seeking
a better quality of health and life.

INTRODUCTION

Usually when people hear about 'keeping fit' all they think about are expensive devices and so many visits to the gym. Sometimes, having to make the frequent visits to the gym can be stressful, time consuming and more often than not, is one of the greatest deterrents.

This simple book documents straight forward steps that you can follow to attain your fitness goals without having to spend huge bills on a personal trainer, a nutritionist, gym tickets, expensive equipment and the several other things that you can think of. Staying healthy should be a primary concern for everybody. It is all in the simple lifestyle that you lead every day, and this book aims to simplify the complex processes to it.

CHAPTER 1

WHY KEEP FIT?

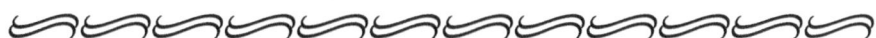

The predominant reason why most people draw up fitness goals is so they can look at their bodies appreciatively.

Before we go further, I would like you to answer these self-motivating questions that have helped a lot of people live the life they dared to imagine.

"How do you see yourself?"

"Do you sometimes wish you could devote some time into caring for yourself, but simply end up berating yourself every day because you know you can do better?"

A lot of people have embarked on a lifestyle of keeping fit just because they want to appreciate the image they see whenever they catch a glimpse of themselves in a mirror. It is important to accept your body and love yourself genuinely. Research shows that it boosts self-confidence.

If you want it, you have to challenge yourself to it. You might start slow, but you have to aim to be better until you get to where you would like to be. Set goals for yourself and walk yourself towards achieving them. Setting fitness goals and aiming to achieve them requires discipline, with calculated and conscious efforts, you can attain them. You do not have to wait until you have all the resources you can picture in your head, you just have to make do with what you have because more often than not, it is more than enough. What is more common is the habit of making excuses instead of finding ways to achieve our desires. Every little input goes a long way. Work with what you have and you will be surprised at how much you can achieve. The most important part however, is to remember to set goals that are realistic. As soon as you are convinced within you that your dreams are attainable, go for them and never feel the need to relent.

If you see the need to shed some weight, do not restrict yourself. You can do it, everybody can.

The sedentary lifestyle predisposes people to several diseases and associated ailments.

It does not matter how busy we think we are, our health should always be our greatest priority. Like the popular adage goes "Health is wealth", I strongly believe that living a good life is the reason why we even work so hard. The moment you let other aspects of your life come in the way of a healthy lifestyle, then you just greatly misinterpreted your priorities and there will be huge consequences sooner or later.

When you cannot keep a good balance between all the aspects of your life, it becomes a problem. I like to believe that health is the most supreme of every aspect there is, thus it should be prioritized over every other.

The World Health Organization describes being healthy as:

A state of complete physical, mental and social well-being, and not merely the absence of disease or infirmity.

Keeping fit does not only give you physical power, it gives you mental power, as well as confidence. It helps you see yourself as a strong individual and also equips you to become one.

Taking care of yourself gives you the strength and the ability to deal with all the other aspects of your life. To decrease the risk of falling sick, and losing out on the very things that we channel our energy and time to, we have to learn to keep our health needs at the forefront of our primary needs, otherwise we risk losing even more time, energy and other resources.

We may not really understand how deteriorated our system becomes every day we fail to discontinue with the constant neglect because it is not visible without clear signs and symptoms that indicate disorders, thus it is highly expedient that we devote more time into caring about our health. We must not wait till we experience complications from living a sedentary lifestyle before we try to curtail it.

Amongst the several things our body requires to function properly, physical activity is the most commonly neglected one.

Overweight and obesity are major risk factors for several health conditions. They include: cardiovascular diseases, type

2 diabetes mellitus, musculoskeletal disorders, cancer, sleep disturbances, arthritis, etc.

Underweight people are not left out either. They are susceptible to immune related problems, musculoskeletal disorders, hypothermia, to mention but a few.

Staying healthy is the optimal thing to do - Identify your limitations and try to improve on them.

CHAPTER 2

A FEW BASICS

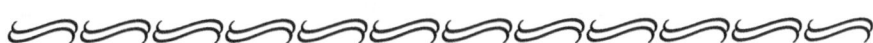

DEFINING YOUR NEEDS

The first step at achieving any set out goal is understanding what it is you want to achieve and why you consider it important. With regards to your health, this should depend on your health status, body composition and preferences. I strongly recommend that you always make your health status the greatest determinant. There is no need trying to get on a certain look just because you think that is what is ideal for you, irrespective of the health consequences. If it is not healthy, it is not the best option. The moment you check your body mass index (BMI) and you realize that it is not within the optimal range, you have a task to work on it. This should determine if you should be losing or gaining weight.

The Body Mass Index is the most common and easiest way to check for weight disorders. It helps point the individual in the right direction. To measure it:

- Check your height in meters
- Check your weight in kilograms

- Then calculate

Height (M²) ÷ Weight (kg)

(Height in meters multiplied by 2 and then divided by the weight in kilograms)

The normal range for adults should be between 18.5 – 24.9.

Below 18.5 indicates an underweight condition, while overweight cases are recorded for figures ranging from 25 -29.9. From 30 and above, we can diagnose cases of obesity.

For overweight people, it is also important to ascertain the level of risk that you are exposed to.

It is important to note that the BMI does not distinguish between the weight from muscles, bones, fats and water. It is important to ascertain where most of the weight is coming from. Your greatest concern is with the weight accrued from fats. Fats will clog your internal organs and impair the functional systems.

Another limitation with the BMI method is that it does not show precisely the location of the fats. Abdominal obesity which is basically fat deposited on your upper body (especially around your abdomen) poses an increased risk to the complications that comes with overweight/obesity.

Thus to get precise results, other methods have been used to better ascertain people who are in danger of this metabolic issue. These kinds of measurements will try to exclude the misleading results from the muscular mass and water weight while concentrating on the fat mass.

They include:

- **Waist to hip ratio:**

This method is very reliable for checking for the risk of abdominal obesity.

The waist to hip ratio is a technique that measures the ratio of the upper body in relation to the lower.

How to check your Waist to Hip Ratio (WHR):

Stand with your feet close to each other. With a measuring tape, take the surround measurement of:

1. Your hips - At its widest part.
2. Your waist - About 1 inch just above the belly button

Take the measurement of the waist at the end of inspiration to get accurate values.

Then calculate: waist surround measurement ÷ hip surround measurement

The resulting value is the waist to hip ratio. Values above 0.90 for males and 0.85 for females indicate abdominal obesity.

- **Specific surround measurements:**

Using a tape measurement, the surround measurements of different parts of the body can be measured and monitored for any visible improvements e.g thighs, abdomen and arms.

The abdominal surround measurement is particularly important because it can also be used as a measure for diagnosing abdominal obesity. Values higher than 89cm in females and 102cm in males signify overweight conditions.

- **Skin fold measurements:**

Using skin calipers, the adipose tissue in different parts of the body can be measured for an estimation of the body fat. The standard sites that are measured include: subscapular skinfold, triceps skinfold, biceps skinfold, abdominal skinfold, anterior thigh skinfold and Supraspinale skinfold.

The sum of each of these sites is then measured and the results are derived and monitored.

The skin fold measurements is a little bit complicated than the other two methods, for people who would like to avoid the technicalities that come with the skin fold measurement processes, the other two methods should be just enough.

IDENTIFYING FOODS

The human body needs food to function. When it comes to food, it should not be the same thing for everybody. You should particularly choose what suits you depending on your needs. Your food plays a very major role in your overall outlook and state of health.

Try to understand the need to and how to choose the right foods for your body. It is usually the reason why people subscribe to nutritionists. If you do not want to use one, then you have to be ready to put in the efforts yourself. This involves taking the time to read and research about different foods. Always remember to make healthy choices. But to be able to make healthy choices, you have to know which foods are healthy. Spend time to talk to someone that knows, read books and try to do your own research.

Sometimes, you might want to eat whatever you like, but you have to understand how this will affect you. If you plan and understand the kinds of food tailored exactly to fit your needs, overtime you will not have any problem choosing healthy foods over anything else that you might be craving.

It will become your habit. In this case, eating healthy is the regular habit and this should be the primary aim for everyone.

COUNTING CALORIES

Every food has an energy value and this is calculated in (kilo) calories. You should get familiar with this to understand your energy needs. A simple calorie counter will help you check your daily caloric intake.

Every time you pick up a packaged food, the energy value is displayed somewhere to help you calculate your caloric intake and inform you on how much the food can spike your blood glucose. This is referred to as the glycemic index.

For whole foods, you have to figure this out by yourself. Fortunately, there are so many options available on the web to make this a lot easier.

Use a calorie counter as much as you can to calculate the energy levels in everything you consume. If you use this tool continuously, overtime, you would not have to always check it, because you will become well acquainted with what to expect.

It is important to understand that for processed foods e.g. packaged chips, the calories are not the same. The calories in processed foods do not need so much time to be broken down like the ones from whole foods. They are 'fast sugars'. They act rapidly to provide quick energy. What this means is that they can easily get you fat if you concentrate on these kinds of dietary sources, thus, it is necessary to pay attention to choosing your foods wisely.

CHOOSING EXERCISES

There are so many forms of exercises and sporting activities that can help you move your body ideally. Everybody needs some form of physical activity. It is not restricted to people trying to lose weight alone. However, choosing the right kind of activity depends on your body needs. A person that is trying to conserve energy for example, has to engage in those kinds of activities that will not induce weight loss. And for those trying to lose weight, there are several activities that can help to expend the excess energy that you could not help acquiring.

It is always good to not starve yourself, rather look for ways to expend the excess calories. Eat healthily and when you need to expend some calories, engage your body in physical activities while aiming to be physically fit and healthy.

For better understanding, it is important to define and distinguish between the terms physical activity, exercise and physical fitness.

> PHYSICAL ACTIVITY: Bodily movement that is produced by the contraction of skeletal muscles which acts to substantially use up energy.

> EXERCISE: A structured and planned type of physical activity with repetitive bodily movement, done to improve and maintain the

components of physical fitness. For example, in the case of overweight/obese people, it is one of the integral parts of a good weight management program.

PHYSICAL FITNESS: Is generally defined as a set of abilities that an individual possesses in order to be able to perform specific types of activities effectively. It is modifiable and this can be done with the help of exercise.

SHOULD YOU GAIN WEIGHT OR LOSE IT?

This is an important question every individual with weight disorders should consider. If you are underweight, then you are trying to add and not lose; and if you are overweight, you should be losing and not adding. It is important that you understand this and keep it in mind because people constantly make the mistake of embarking on a task that is the direct opposite of what their body requires. You are doing your body more harm than good when you neglect what your body needs for what you want. Contrary to what the society wants us to believe, an underweight person has a weight disorder just like an overweight person does. None is better. They are both health disorders. The best line of action is to remedy the disorder. To manage these health disorders, you have to understand the relationship between the food you take (caloric intake) and the amount of physical activity you undergo every day (caloric expenditure). The way you see your body is as a result of the ratio of your caloric intake and caloric expenditure.

BASAL METABOLIC RATE

To lose or add weight, first you have to define your Basal Metabolic Rate (BMR).

This refers to the amount of energy your body uses up at rest. The body needs to expend a certain amount of energy just to function daily. This rate is different for different people and it has a huge role to play in the amount of fats you retain every day.

Using the Harris – Benedict formula, we can calculate the BMR thus:

For females:

655 + (4.3 x your weight in pounds) + (4.7 x your height in inches) - (4.7 x your age)

For males:

66 + (6.3 x your weight in pounds) + (12.9 x your height in inches) - (6.8 X your age)

If you are trying to lose weight, you have to take in less calories than your BMR requires and if you are trying to add, you have to make sure that you have more than enough.

If you are trying to gain weight, then you need to gain more calories (dietary intake), while expending less (conserving energy); and if you are trying to lose, you want to do the direct opposite; expend more (physical activity), gain less (less calorie consumption).

Gaining weight is simply via food consumption and expending is by physical activity. This is as simple as you read it; it is not complicated at all.

People that are trying to lose weight should not be conserving energy. Interestingly, that is what happens when you eat and just laze around.

CHAPTER 3

LOSING WEIGHT

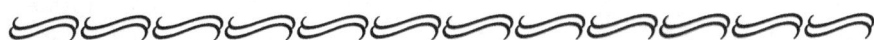

Losing weight requires modifications in two principal aspects: Nutrition and lifestyle.

Remember the weight ratio that I mentioned earlier? We will be applying it practically now. Due to genetics, some people tend to retain a lot of fats than others, but physical activity can function to not only help expend excess fats, but also increase the basal metabolic rate.

Levine et al conducted a research to explain the thermogenesis of the body as it helps to use up energy. With this study, these researchers tried to categorize the thermogenesis that occurs via physical activity as follows:

- Volitional exercise: These kinds of activities include sports, fitness related activities and exercises.
- Non – exercise activity thermogenesis: This one has to do with more regular activities of daily living. Examples include: Nodding the head, maintaining a good posture, fidgeting and more spontaneous muscle contractions.

This research involved monitoring people who all ate the same meals and were locked up in a laboratory for two months without active exercising. It was noted that some of them could not just sit still for hours. Their bodies were constantly making some sort of inherent movements unconsciously. These subjects were monitored for a period of two months, during which it was discovered that the category of subjects who just could not sit still did not gain weight unlike the others and they also had a higher BMR. Dr. Jensen, one of the collaborators in the study explained the reason to be a consequence of the Non-exercise Activity Thermogenesis (NEAT). He also explained via this study that when people sit for hours, the electrical activity in their muscles drop, causing an array of harmful metabolic effects. The rate at which they burn calories drop to about one per minute and the enzymes responsible for breaking down fats are also reduced. This study in the long run confirms the effectiveness of an active lifestyle in propagating increased fat metabolism.

To lose weight you need to eat foods that offer minimal calories while engaging in activities that will make you lose excess calories. This is the basis of every weight loss program. This is the reason why you go to the gym and the reason why people choose the option of starving themselves.

This brings me to talk about the negative aspects of starvation. Even though starving helps cut down on the amount of calories you ingest, it sure does a lot of harm. The body uses nutrients from food to function effectively. The body needs some nutrients specifically on a daily basis, without which we will see series of deficiency syndromes (depending on the nutrient that is lacking). These nutrients that the body cannot do without are referred to as 'essential nutrients'.

Nutrients are described as essential because:

1. They play important roles in the body that must not be neglected.
2. They cannot be produced by the body or in the adequate amount that the body requires.

3. They are raw materials for producing other nutrients.

These essential nutrients are important for everyone.

They include:

- Certain fatty acids: If you choose good fat sources and not take too much of them, you do not have to worry about your weight loss goals. Fatty acids are obtained from fat sources. Examples of good sources include: olive oil, canola oil, fish, sunflower oil, etc.

- Certain amino acids: Proteins are important building blocks for the body. They can help in your weight loss goals by keeping your tummy full while adding fewer calories. Amino acids are the by-products of protein. Sources include: seafood, dairy products, lean cuts of meat, vegetable protein and eggs.

- Some minerals: Minerals cannot be produced by the body, thus they must be supplied to the body through nutrition. They have different functions ranging from forming the structure of different parts of the body to regulating important pathways within the body. They are divided into the macro and micro minerals. The 'macro elements' are those required by the body in large quantities while the 'micro elements' are also referred to as the 'trace elements', because they are needed in very small amounts.

The macro elements include: Sodium, potassium, chloride, calcium, magnesium, phosphorus and sulfur. The trace elements include: zinc, iron, copper, manganese, fluoride, iodine and molybdenum.

These minerals have different sources but they are more frequently obtained from vegetables, fruits, seafood, dairy products, eggs, whole grains and nuts.

- Vitamins: Just like the minerals, vitamins are those nutrients that do not supply calories but are also very relevant for a functioning body. They are usually needed in small quantities.

They are grouped into two: fat soluble vitamins and the water soluble vitamins.

The fat soluble vitamins are vitamins that are only soluble in fats. They are Vitamins A, D, E and K.

The water soluble vitamins are those that are soluble in water. They include vitamin C and vitamin B-complex.

The different vitamins can be obtained from a variety of sources which include: vegetables, fruits, cereal, liver, dairy products, whole grains and nuts.

A few helpful 'dos and do nots':

1. Do not spend on dieting pills

Most of them do not work. Well, you might say there is one that does. But how many will you try until you find that one? Do you understand the amount of damage you expose yourself to by ingesting these chemicals? The one you might think actually works, because it helps you achieve your goal of losing weight might be very harmful to your overall health. It is not worth the risk at all. Stick to natural remedies and give it some time and patience.

2. Eat less

Cut out the indulgences. Never overeat. You will need to work harder to expend the excess calories. It is much easier for fat people to gain weight than it is for them to lose it. Avoiding it is much safer. Do not starve, rather eat only when you are hungry and always choose healthy options. The process of being hungry is a physiological response which informs you that your cells need food, use it effectively.

The worst thing you can do to yourself is to binge eat without control. Here is a trick that most people miss. No matter the kind of food you eat, it does not matter if you are eating just veggies and fruits, overfeeding will still have consequences. Eat until the point where you are just satisfied and stop before you feel really full. You can always go back and eat again when you do feel hungry. Do not try to take in everything in one go. Make it a habit to stay away from stuffing yourself up.

You might think a few days of indulging would not harm you so much if you try to lose the excess calories after, but you are wrong; apart from having to worry about the accumulated calories, you have to understand that the walls of your stomach are made of smooth muscles which have elastin as its main component. Elastin is a type of fiber that works just like the name suggests, 'elastic'. It expands when stretched. The moment you fill it up to its limit, it becomes stretched and continues to expand. This means that you will succeed in increasing the capacity of your stomach and this will influence the amount of food you eat every day, as it will take more amounts to get you to the point of satisfaction.

Discipline yourself and no matter where you find yourself, always follow this simple principle.

3. Introduce fiber into your meals

The role of fiber in this case will be to prolong the process of digestion and absorption, since it usually takes longer to digest these food sources. Your body will require more time to break the food down, which will in turn delay the time for you to feel hungry.

Some sources of fiber include: vegetables, fruits, whole grains, etc.

These can serve as very good options for snacking as well.

4. Use water as a filler

I have also noticed over time that most fat people have the tendency of sensing hunger than normal. This is usually more of a psychological issue. A smart way to resolve this is to plan your meals. Make a mental note of when you should be having each meal to avoid eating more than necessary and if you feel the need to eat before then, use water as a filler. Water does not possess any caloric content which makes it the perfect filler. Also, if you want to have little portions of food but tend to eat a lot before you reach the point of satisfaction, start by drinking water. This will give you very little room to put food, thereby helping to regulate the caloric intake. Remember, do not starve yourself!

5. Maximize what you have

Run, jog, walk your dog, ride a bicycle, take it to the streets; anything to help you increase your physical activity levels. These are simple activities that do not require you to spend, but can help you burn the excess calories. Make the most of them.

6. Cut the sleeping and lazing around time

Get busy! Instead of sleeping around at home, work. It will really help you check the cravings. Find some great activities that can keep you busy instead of lazing around the house, eating and sleeping.

7. Plan a schedule

Try to plan a time routine and stick to it. With this you can choose exercises that permit you to stay within the comfort of your home. The options are enormous e.g. skipping, jogging, brisk walking. The most important aspect is to be consistent.

The greatest advantage of planning a simple routine is that after a while your body gets accustomed to it. Try to keep it regular, especially the timing because it works better. A person that trains every morning is definitely at a greater advantage of attaining their goals than someone who does it whenever they feel like. The reason is because after a while, their body will try to adapt to this timing and will in turn initiate a response to prepare the body for the activity prior to the time of the scheduled workout. This indeed is an added advantage.

8. Try some sporting activities

It does not have to be hectic for it to work. This is what I try to explain every time I get the chance. Just have fun while at it.

Fall back on those outdoor games you used to embark on as a child. It does not hurt at all to play. I believe everybody has a certain sport that they love, use it to your advantage. You are looking for any opportunity to lose some weight. Trying your favorite sporting activity will give you a chance to lose it over something you enjoy doing. You do not have any? Choose one, it is pretty easy. All you need is to develop the interest for it.

You would be so surprised how easy and how much fun it is to just dance. I believe everybody can dance. It is as easy as just moving your body to your favorite kind of music. You can use it for cardio fitness, weight loss, mobility training, etc. (depending on how you engage it). For weight loss, always remember to aim for long durations. You do not need to be a great dancer for this to be effective. All you want is the opportunity to move your body for a considerable long period of time, enough to target your fat stores.

Swimming is another good option for instance.

9. Plan and prepare your meals before hand

Preparing your meal before time gives you the room to source for the best available options. This will help limit the number of times that you will try to just grab something to satisfy your hunger. Chances are that usually when you are extremely hungry and you decide to grab whatever is available, it will not be the best choice like if you had enough time to prepare for it. The idea is to try to avoid such situations by planning ahead.

10. Improve your lifestyle

You might not have all the time every day to put in a good workout, but if you put in some great efforts, they will go a long way. It is all in the simple things you do every day e.g. using the stairs instead of the elevator. It could be a little time consuming if you have to walk to work/school instead of driving for instance, but you have to plan your time well and dedicate some time into making it work.

Eliminate the drinking, the smoking, the starving, the binge eating and the many other unhealthy lifestyles that you can think of.

In summary:

- Identify the cause and tackle it
- Engage in structured physical activities
- Learn to choose your foods right
- Control your cravings, but eat when you are hungry
- Eat smaller portions of food

And most importantly, plan a simple but healthy overall lifestyle. Nothing too complicated, nothing too fancy or demanding; just be more attentive to your body.

CHAPTER 4

GAINING WEIGHT

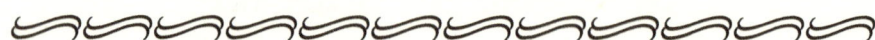

It is rather interesting how most people overlook the phrase 'healthy does not mean skinny'. There are so many underweight people who believe they are perfect, just because they are skinny.

You turn to the web and you see a thousand ideas and people airing concerns on how to lose weight and almost nothing on gaining weight. Most people do not remember that there are also lots of people trying to gain some reasonable amount of weight just as much as we have those trying to lose them. It might just be someone that noticed that he/she is a little skinny and needs to modify their look, or someone who understands the implications of not being within the healthy weight range. It might even be someone that just recovered from a health condition with severe muscle wasting. The point is, never forget that even though obesity has turned out to be a huge epidemic, there are also people trying to find good ways to gain some weight.

The reason people do not bother, I am sure is because we tend to easily put on weight unconsciously by unhealthy life choices. And I am sure right now, a lot of you are already thinking "of course, I know how to add weight if I want to". You might have even considered skipping this part because you think it is not important to you. If you just thought about all the unhealthy ways of adding weight e.g. binging on junk foods, then you need to concentrate on this part more. What is the point of adding some weight, looking prettier in your dress and jeopardizing your health in the process?

Staying healthy should always be your greatest goal and I will not suggest anything that jeopardizes that in any regard. Whenever you are thinking of gaining weight, always think about regular, well-balanced and nutritious diets. A well balanced diet includes all the classes of food in their optimal proportions.

They include:

- Carbohydrates

- Proteins

- Fats

- Vitamins

- Minerals

- Water

These are the basic classes of foods.

Carbohydrates, fats and protein are those that provide the body with calories. The other nutrients are also important in the body because they play vital functions. Carbohydrate is the immediate source of energy and when that is not available, the body utilizes the fats. When that is also exhausted, the protein stores are then targeted. The depletion of the protein stores will lead to muscle wasting.

Choose healthy, energy dense foods, especially those that offer more than one nutrient. A typical example is seafood. You can have protein, fats and different minerals packed into a small serving of fish. If you are someone that cannot eat a lot, this is quite beneficial. Also, look for creative ways you can add more calories in each serving, e.g. adding cheese to pasta, eggs to mashed potatoes, rich oils to soups, the possibilities are endless and it is all up to your creativity.

Whatever you do, do not buy into the idea that slim people need not exercise. Engaging in useful physical activities is an essential for everyone. Choose exercises that do not induce weight loss, but do not completely abstain from exercising. As a matter of fact, some exercises will help build up your muscle and make you look more toned and healthy.

In Summary:

- Identify the cause and curtail it
- Eat regularly to provide your body with enough energy to undergo its activity.
- Always remember to choose good sources, and use healthy serving and cooking options.
- Do not give your body room to turn to your stored energy. Choose exercises that suit this preference.

CHAPTER 5

BUILDING BULK

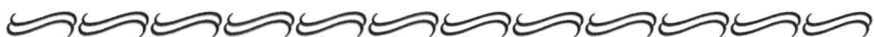

Choosing activities that help to build muscles can be quite rewarding. For those that are skinny, building up your muscle will help increase its diameter and make you look healthier. Everybody, including people that are trying to lose weight need to learn how to train their muscles. In this case, the goal should be to replace the fat mass with muscle, otherwise, when you cut down the fat mass, all that will be left underneath will be a thin layer of subcutaneous tissue and flabby muscles. Also, the bigger the muscles, the more energy you will use up while performing activities of daily living (and other activities).

The need to introduce resistance training into your workouts cannot be over emphasized. With resistance training you can induce muscle growth as well as muscle strengthening.

For muscle growth, you will need to start with lifting loads that appear to be heavy. Heavy weight lifting will induce muscle growth. This will result in few repetitions which allow your muscle to keep growing to adapt to it. You can keep improving on your progressions with time, by increasing the load. When you have reached your desired size, you can then start building strength.

For muscle strengthening, you will need to adopt an absolutely different strategy. Light weights with more repetitions will help to strengthen the muscles. For this, you will need to concentrate more on the number of repetitions. More repetitions will work to keep the muscle looking firm and toned.

I must also add that these are not as isolated as it seems. Understanding how to speed things up functions to help you focus your efforts on your specific goals.

How to incorporate resistance training into your workout:

- Use your body weight

One great benefit of going to the gym is that you can find various equipment for resistance training, but the good news is that you can always improvise. The first source of load you should always think about is your body weight. If you use the right techniques, you should be able to achieve great results just by redirecting your body weight to different parts of your body through the way you position your body. Work with gravity and find positions where more force is exerted at the sections you are targeting. When you are using your body weight for resistance training, it is more effective when you take things slowly. Take your time with every move as opposed to going fast. You also want to ensure that you direct the movements against the direction of the gravitational force to be able to engage the load from your body weight maximally.

• Isometric contractions

This can also be referred to as 'static contractions'. This can be achieved by contracting and restricting the targeted part of the body with objects or by resistance from another person. A typical example is holding down a squatting position to exert contractions on the lower region of the body.

- Lift weights

This is achieved by lifting external load. You can get your own dumbbells or improvise by lifting heavy objects around the house, but take note of how to incorporate progressions if your aim is to induce muscle growth. To increase your progression you should keep increasing the load.

- Use elastic bands

Pulling on tight elastic bands also produce a resistive force on the targeted part of the body. Again, you have to pay attention to the progression. In this case, keep reducing the length of the band and also progress to thicker band options.

A few examples of workouts for resistance training include:

Hands - Pull on an elastic band

Legs - Squats

Shoulders - Press ups

Trunk - Pull ups

Abdominals – Crunches

If you do not want to look bulky, remember to include exercises that help you elongate your muscles after building them up. Examples include Pilates and yoga.

CHAPTER 6

ARE YOU WORKING HARD BUT NOT SEEING RESULTS?

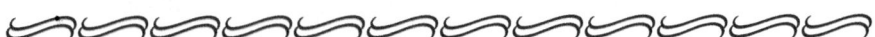

The first thing to consider when trying to achieve your goals is to identify those factors that act as deterrents. It is important to understand the cause of every weight disorder to effectively tackle it. For instance, obesity that is as a consequence of alcoholism will require an alcohol cessation intervention within the weight loss program for it to be effective. An overall lifestyle assessment is recommended as the first line of solution for every weight management program.

Also, your dietary intake is the greatest determinant of the way your body pans out. Some people think they can eat just about anything and work it out at the gym. To lose one pound of fat, you have to expend 3500 calories. Think about the fact that your regular burgers from most of these fast food joints have about 1000 – 1500 calories (or even more), depending. And this is what you ingest in just one sitting and that means that is not all you would be eating for the day because you are definitely going to eat some more, except you want to starve for the rest of the day. That is a consequence of ill planning because using up all those excess calories will require a whole lot of exercising. How often do you even exercise or have time to exercise? So what do you think happened to the rest of those excess calories you could not use up? The answer is pretty straight forward - Your body retained them as fat stores.

That simply explains the bugging issue "I am working out but I do not see any changes". There will be no changes if you do not find a way to expend more and retain less. If you finish a simple workout and then go ahead to binge on food that is even more than the calories you managed to lose during your workout, the desired changes will not be effected.

Let us look at it practically:

> For example, if you want to lose 1 pound in 2 weeks
>
> 1 pound = 3500 kcal (454 grams, 0.454 kilograms)
>
> 3500 ÷ 14 = 250

If you stick to losing 250 calories daily, at the end of two weeks you would have lost 1 pound.

Also, you have to be sure that your aerobic workout is effective to target your fat stores. Aim for moderate intensities that last up to an average of 30 – 45 minutes for effective results.

And to address "I am trying to add weight and nothing is showing."

You have to do the complete opposite. Firstly, you have to understand that starving and eating whenever you feel like might result in your body trying to deplete your fat stores. Do not think that you can eat well today and starve tomorrow and that will just be enough. You have to learn to keep it regular. The idea is to stick to keeping supposed 'quick fixes' as habits.

When you starve, your body begins to use up stored up energy because there is no ready supply of energy. This will only result in leaner muscles. What you want to do is to retain enough energy by always giving your body an immediate and steady supply of energy. To remedy this, eat frequently and do not give your body room to turn to the reserves.

It is rather rampant – albeit a huge mistake – to see people skipping breakfast. Breakfast is very important. Remember that you usually have a very long period of time where you had to fast (the whole time you were asleep at night), basically it is somewhat like starving, and then you wake up in the morning and decide to starve some more?

It might not be very easy for people with very busy schedules, but all you might need would be to wake up a bit earlier than usual and make it a habit to always supply your body the required energy to work with, before running out of your house.

Let us look at our calculations again:

> This time, let's assume that you want to add 1 pound in 1 week.
>
> You will simply need to eat an excess of 500 calories daily (That is what you should retain after all daily activities)
>
> 500 x 7 = 3500

If you remember from our calculations, 1 pound consists of 3500 calories

Now, I am sure you understand how important it is to understand your BMR before embarking on creating a strategy to achieve your fitness goals.

Another important aspect is to look for appropriate ways to measure your progress. Some people try to measure how well their efforts are paying off by evaluating themselves using the mental picture they have created for themselves as the yardstick. This will lead to a negative perception of the realities. This will either result in a withdrawal response or make you look for unrealistic ways to attain your goals speedily. Sometimes, your mirror might not give you a true representation of your results or you may be blinded by focusing on what you want to see. That is, you look at yourself and you are blinded by the fact that you do not look half as what you would want to look like, and because of this you are not able to notice the changes that your hard-work has been able to effect. You need to get rid of that mental picture of who you want to look like and get good measuring tools instead. Try a measuring tape or a weighing scale and you will see that if you are actually putting in the effort, then there will always be results. It might not be very significant initially, but you have to pay attention to be able to notice the very little steps that contribute to the bigger picture. This is very important. Being able to see the result of your efforts, no matter how little it might seem, would make you want to dedicate more time into being consistent with what you are doing, because you already know that it would pay off.

Do not forget that keeping fit requires a lot of calculated moves. It is all about creativity and determination. Set your goal, make a good plan and find those factors that will help you stick to it.

CHAPTER 7

WORKING WITH
YOUR MINDSET

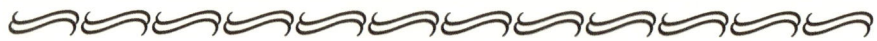

Whenever you embark on anything new, there is always the possibility of letting go to settle for those things you are already conversant with and that is why you always need loads and loads of motivation. Your psychology plays a very essential role when it comes to achieving desired goals.

Here are a few helpful tips:

- Social help

Interacting with the right kind of people; people that share a common interest with you or understand your struggles can be quite beneficial. Join forums, seek ideas, learn from other people, while aiming to support and motivate each other. You can always use the help of a friend, who will in turn be very appreciative of your company. The best part is the impact of collective efforts, which will help make individual efforts almost unrecognizable. You will realize that the whole tension is lifted off when you see others that are even more passionate about their goals than you are. The encouragement you seem to gain from interacting with others goes a long way in helping you actualize your goals with less difficulty.

However, you must understand that we all have different goals and needs. Choosing somebody whose needs are so far apart from yours can lead to a negative perception of yourself or desires. I strongly recommend that you pay attention to the kind of opinions you subscribe to. It should be that of people who share a similar interest with you or have your best interest at heart. Try to understand how to eliminate pressure that may stem from interacting with other people that have a different set of goals and aspirations than yours.

- Music

Spend time and make a good collection of great songs for your long workouts, it goes a long way. Choose fast paced songs and avoid songs that will dampen your mood. Also, try to choose songs with very motivational lyrics. Just imagine hearing words like "yes, you can do it" on a day when you feel extremely frustrated. Music is invigorating; it is almost incredible how magical it can be.

- Switch things up

When it comes to working out, you have to be very innovative and creative, otherwise it might become boring. Always switch it up when it feels like you have been doing the same thing over and over again. You will feel more excitement when you have to try something new and this can boost positive energy and also prevent your body from getting too adapted to the training. When your body gets adapted to your routine, you hit a plateau which makes it hard to effect any progressions. Always try to see how you can introduce something new and interesting, and also remember to add some elements of fun to it. Something exciting, something that wants to make you do it over and over again without feeling the stress or making you feel like you are compelled to it.

- Do not overtrain

Introduce rest periods so you do not become fatigued. Do not allow the pressure to get everything in one attempt overshadow the need for a well-structured plan. Try to relax and think more about long term goals instead of rapid ones.

- Choose comfortable outfits

Nothing will get you easily fatigued like a restricting outfit. It is bad when your lack of motivation comes from something as basic as choosing an outfit. Invest in something convenient.

These handy tips can make a whole lot of difference.

CHAPTER 8

A GREAT WORKOUT PLAN

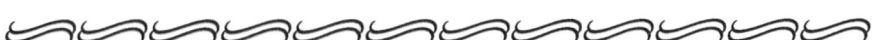

A great workout plan begins with choosing the best form of exercise that suits your needs. Remember to put into consideration the mode of exercise and the duration. For a workout that is targeted at weight loss, the process should last up to 30-45 minutes for you to be able to engage your fat stores effectively. A 5-minute workout for instance, will use your glucose stores and not your fat stores.

Oxidation of fat occurs during aerobic metabolism. Since oxygen does not increase immediately at the onset of the exercise, this part of the exercise is anaerobic (not aerobic). Under anaerobic conditions, carbohydrates are usually the most readily source of energy utilized.

The energy sources for the body are as follows:

- Adenosine triphosphate (ATP): This energy phosphate is the energy used by the muscles to perform activities of daily living. The amount of energy found in muscles is relatively small, thus the body needs to resynthesize them through other chemical reactions continuously.

What this means is that any quick action will first involve the use of the ATP stored in the muscles before activating the production of more by other sources when the (quick) energy is being used up.

- Phosphocreatine: This is a very rapid source and it involves only one enzymatic step. In this reaction, this complex amino acid is re-phosphorylated to Adenosine triphosphate (ATP) from Adenosine diphosphate (ADP). Creatine kinase catalyses the reaction to release a phosphate group to ADP so that ATP can be produced.

- Glycolysis

When you perform continuous strenuous activities, there is compensation through excessive ventilation by the individual which will result in increased oxygen consumption, thus the aerobic system is triggered. The aerobic workout is enabled by energy from this aerobic system. Glycolysis involves a series of chemical reactions catalyzed by different enzymes responsible for the degradation of carbohydrate to smaller substrates for energy production. This starts off the aerobic system. The process however begins with anaerobic metabolism. In the presence of oxygen, pyruvate is further decarboxylated to acetyl - coA which is a substrate for the Kreb's cycle. The aerobic system consists of the the Kreb's cycle (including the aerobic part of glycolysis) and Beta oxidation of fat. In the absence of oxygen, the pyruvate will be converted to lactate instead and stored in the muscles.

To make things even clearer, let us look at the difference between the short term, high intensity exercise and the long term, low to moderate intensity exercise.

Short term, high intensity exercise: (5-60 seconds)

When a muscular activity is about 5 seconds or lower than 5 seconds, the energy required to perform this activity is from the adenosine triphosphate – Creatine Phosphate (ATP-CP) system. When exercises last longer than this period, there will be a gradual shift from the energy supplied by the ATP-CP system to the anaerobic part of the glycolytic pathway.

Exercises that last up to 45 seconds will use a combination of the ATP-CP system and the anaerobic parts of glycolysis. Exercises that last longer will trigger a progression to the aerobic system. The anaerobic sources will make about 70% while the remaining 30% will be completed by the aerobic metabolism. The energy used up by this system is mostly that of carbohydrate stored up in the form of glycogen in the muscle, converted to glucose and used to produce energy for the work.

Long term, low - moderate intensity exercise: (10 – 60 minutes)

Oxygen consumption (Vo_2) can be maintained during 10 – 60 minutes of low and moderate intensity exercise. During this period, the aerobic oxidative phosphorylation occurs. There is a gradual shift from the use of carbohydrate substrates to that of fats, thus, to be able to target these fat stores, low intensity to moderate exercises should be used. These sorts of exercises will utilize oxygen to produce more ATPs from fats. This is what sustains the workouts to last even longer. Without adequate oxygen, it is necessary to stop the workout. The physiological response would be when you find yourself gasping for breath.

It is also important to note that if you have your work-out in the morning before having your breakfast, this period of being able to target your fat stores will greatly decrease, whereas in the evening after you have had so many meals, it will take more time to use up the readily available energy source before heading to your fat stores. The time of the day is another factor that you should pay attention to. Use this to adjust the duration of your exercise.

Finally, here is a simple structure of what a simple workout plan should be made of:

1. Warm up session – About 2-5 minutes
   Introduce mild movements to get your system ready. A few stretching techniques can be included here to engage the muscles slowly.

2. The main exercise – 10-40 minutes

   These can include: dance aerobics, running, resistance training, cycling, hiking, playing football, rowing, swimming, etc.

   Choose something that works for your needs.

   Try to introduce rest periods in between, during which you can catch a breather and drink some water to prevent dehydration and fatigue.

3. Cool down period - About 2-5 minutes

   Here you gradually lower the tempo of the exercise routine as opposed to stopping abruptly. You do not want to feel like everything in you just collapsed. Again, this can include stretching exercises and mild movements. The idea is to take it from moderate back to low before gradually ending your session.

CHAPTER 9

CLEARING SOME MYTHS

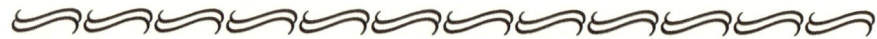

Having to talk to people trying to lose weight, I noticed something that was almost always inevitable with most of them – they always had one misconception or the other. It is important that you understand that when you stick to these rules that are not logical, you jeopardize your chances of finding suitable programs that should help you achieve your goals, hence the need to address them. Here are a few interesting ones that have been very frequently mentioned:

1. "Always eat dinner before 8pm"

You might have heard this if you join a fitness forum. The reason people say this is not just based on the time itself, rather they try to estimate the time until you go to bed. When you sleep off immediately after your meal, you slow down the digestion process which reduces your fat burning process and your body retains most of the food. It takes about 2-3 hours for the food to be digested (depending on the kind of food you had), so it is important to think about giving yourself this kind of time between after having your dinner and going to bed. This effort is absolutely futile if you eat until 8pm when you are going to bed immediately after.

2. "Only men should lift weights because it makes women look masculine"

This is not true. To be able to train your muscles to look masculine, you ought to be working out on an extremely professional level (e.g. athletes). Training with weights a couple of times will not give you that masculine look. The reason is because men have large amounts of testosterone and this is what helps to hasten things up. Resistance training helps build your muscle, do not limit yourself. Use light weights and try to incorporate them into your workout routines. The trick is in knowing when to stop. Moderation is key!

3. "You can eat as much as you want as long as you work out before or after"

This also is a very wrong myth. I already talked extensively about this in the preceding chapters. It is very wrong to practice this if you are trying to lose weight. You will really jeopardize your efforts.

(See chapter 3 for more)

4. "Stretching is a big waste of time"

There are still a lot of controversies as to whether stretching helps to prevent injury as people believe or not. Most athletes say it sucks up the energy they would have used for the main task. It is important to note that by stretching before you engage in vigorous exercises, you warm up your muscles and the circulation to sustain the load, especially if your routine will involve swift movements. Also, stretching produces an eccentric force on the muscle. This kind of contraction helps to lengthen your muscle. Thus, stretching helps for flexibility which will help increase the range of motion. This in itself helps to prevent muscle strain and tear. However, it is always important to keep it simple and short otherwise, you might lose energy to carry out the main task. From my personal experience, I can tell the difference with or without stretching. Stretching makes movements a lot easier.

5. "Use energy drinks to help you last longer while exercising"

The moment you use energy drinks during a fat loss workout, the purpose has been defeated already because you will use the fast source of energy instead of depleting your fat stores. When you exercise for a long period, your body switches from using the readily available ATPs present in your muscles to producing them via fat metabolism, when you introduce sugars into your body during your workout, your system recognizes this and cuts down on the long process of breaking down the fats.

It will immediately switch to using the quick glucose you provided.

6. "Exercising is only for overweight people"

At this point, you should already know that this is not true. From the very first chapter, I tried to elaborate on why it is important for everyone to engage in some form of physical activity. Choose the one that suits you best depending on your needs and preferences.

7. "Do not undergo aerobic activities except when you are trying to lose weight"

Aerobic activities are very good for the cardiovascular system. It is wrong not to introduce them into your routines. To initiate weight loss, the key is to keep it long enough. Without the long duration, it is just enough to kick start the cardiovascular system on a faster level thereby enhancing cardio-fitness.

8. "When you are looking for foods with few calories, choose salads"

People make the mistake to think that as long as it is a salad, it is safer than any other choice. Well, there are different kinds of salads and just because it has a few vegetables and fruits does not mean that you should not pay attention to the other contents. Most times, your greatest worry should be the dressing. If only you could calculate the amount of calories in some of those greasy, fatty pastes that cover those veggies, you would realize that your salad is not exactly as safe as you think it is. However, fruits and vegetables have fewer calories compared to so many other nutrient sources, use it to your advantage.

9. "You achieve the best results when you can lose so much weight at the shortest period of time"

According to the American Council of Sports Medicine, the healthy weight loss range is between 1.5lbs - 2lbs per week.

Severe emaciation should serve as an indication for a health disorder and deliberately inducing this is totally misleading. The result is usually a shrinking of the skin and that can be avoided. Follow a healthy process and do not forget that you should always think about your body as a whole whenever you are choosing any remedy for any aspect you are uncomfortable with.

10. "You have to sweat for it to be a good workout"

Letting all that steam and toxin out is definitely a big plus, but it should not be the primary determinant of a good workout. I say this because most people forget to build their workouts in terms of the duration and intensity but rely solely on when their bodies seem to vent the most to determine when they have reached a great intensity. On the other hand, others seem to overtrain because they just cannot feel the evidence of the workout in the form they want to see (that is sweating).

Remember that several factors will contribute to the way your body will react, especially the weather and the kind of clothes you have on. Make a workout plan with well-defined goals and use that instead, this will help you determine your progression a whole lot and not on sweating because that can be very misleading.

CONCLUSION

Conclusively, I would like to advice that you remember to give yourself the maximum attention that it requires, no matter what you do and where you find yourself. The main aim is to look for what applies and works best for you. It is not the same for everyone.

I hope that this book was able to awaken that new desire in you to stay fit and healthy, clear some of your doubts about fitness and equip you on what to do.

REFERENCES

Research for *The Easy Way to Keeping Fit* includes:

1. Barrett, K. E. & Ganong, W.F. (2012). *Ganong's Review of Medical Physiology.* New York, McGraw-Hill Medical.

2. Donnelly, J. E., Blair, S.N., Jakicic, J.M., Manore, M. M., Rankin, J.W., & Smith, B.K. (2009). *American College of Sports Medicine position stand. Appropriate physical activity intervention strategies for weight loss and prevention of weight regain for adults:* Medicine and Science in Sports and Exercise 41(2); 459-471.

3. Ehrman, J.K. (2010). *ACSM's Resource Manual for Guidelines for Exercise Testing and Prescription.* Philadelphia: Wolters Kluwer Health/Lippincott Williams & Wilkins.

4. Goodman, C. C., & Fuller, K.S. (2009). *Pathology: Implications for the physical therapist.* St. Louis, Mo: Saunders/Elsevier.

5. Guyton, C. A., & Hall, J. E. (2011). *Guyton and Hall Textbook of Medical Physiology.* Philadelphia: Elsevier Saunders.

6. Hough, A. (2001). *Physiotherapy in Respiratory Care: An Evidence-Based Approach to Respiratory and Cardiac Management.* Cheltenham: Nelson Thornes.

7. Levine, J. A., Eberhardt, N.L, & Jensen, M.D. (1999). *Role of non-exercise activity thermogenesis in resistance to fat gain in humans.* Science. 283(5399); 212-4.

8. McArdle, W. D., Katch, F.I., & Katch, V.L. (2001). *Exercise Physiology: Energy, nutrition and human performance.* Philadelphia: Lippincott Williams and Wilkins.

9. Postlethwait, J. H. & Hopson, J. L. (2006). *Modern Biology.* Orlando: Holt, Rinehart and Wineston.

10. Wolpert, S. (2007). Dieting Does Not Work, UCLA Researchers Report. *UCLA Newsroom. April, 3.*

11. World Health Organization. (2007). Basic documents. *WHO Media Centre. Geneva, Switzerland.*

12. World Health Organization. (2013). Obesity and overweight Fact sheet N 311. *WHO Media Centre. Geneva, Switzerland.*